Special Education to College:

THE KETRINA STORY

W0017430

"BREAKING THOSE
GLASS CEILINGS."

©KETRINA HAZELL

CONTENTS

Dedication

Dedication

This book is dedicated to parents, caregivers, educators, and anyone who plays a role in serving the youth who need extra support and young people with disabilities or unique needs, and those placed in special education due to having behavioural, learning, or emotional needs. In this book, you will find many answers to questions that you may not have known you had until after reading this, about all of the hardships people with disabilities such as myself have to go through. As a reader, you will understand what it is like for those struggling with their education. I hope that by the end of this book, you will realize that you are not alone. Whether you have a disability or not, if you are a parent with a child with a disability, or even if you are just an individual struggling to get through school, this book is for you.

Limitless Me

It started with an Individualized Education Program (IEP). Medical documents, individual life plans, employment plans, and psychological and psychosocial evaluations were supposed to grant me the life I desired, but this was not always the case. Instead, these documents were used to define me. My IEP gave me the accommodations I needed throughout elementary, middle, high school and college. However, the document also made me look like I was not college-capable, and it gave me no pathway or actions to follow for a smooth transition into adulthood.

My college grade point average (GPA) tried to interpret my intelligence to define what I was intellectually capable of. While compiling all of these documents into a file, I anticipated when I could freely live out my dreams without limitations. I refused to have society, statistics, and data models prove what I was capable of. Did any of these matter as I embarked on the path of —limitless me‖?

Know who you are and not what society expects of you. I am turning the page and just living life to the fullest; disability should not limit me. I am becoming everything I desired to be and hoped for. You are defined by Your passions, Your aspirations, Your story. Let us get started!

When the School System First Began to Have Low Expectations of Me

My name is Ketrina Hazell. I was diagnosed with a disability at nine months old. Doctors had low expectations of what my life could be like having a developmental disability. They told my parents I would never be able to see, hear, talk, walk, or do anything like a "typical child". When I began early intervention, my parents were informed that I had cerebral palsy. Early Intervention was where I started making progress in learning with my teachers and had more development with physical, occupational, and speech therapy. Honestly, I was placed in "special education" because I have a physical disability, classified as a developmental disability. So how did I fit in to become qualified to receive special education classroom support and services? Is it simply because I have used a wheelchair? My disability classification in my Individual Educational Program is Multiple Disabilities. Today, I am wondering what that means. I know I spent time in special education because of my disability, and I could not (and still cannot) move at the same speed as my peers without physical disabilities. I did things slower than others and took the time to process lots of information at once. For example, I had trouble with math for as long as I could remember, but once I was given the tools and assignments in a modified curriculum, excelling beyond did not matter to educators; they were okay with what I knew.

I always dream big despite my disabilities, but over time, growing up, my confidence has shattered on many levels, and so have my dreams.

When I was four or five years old, a school psychologist evaluated me, and because I was timid growing up, I did not appropriately respond to her. She did not even give me a second chance. Finally, she decided I did not know my colors. She recommended that I be placed in a classroom with children considered "mentally retarded" (it is now known as intellectual or developmental disabilities as a better way to define people with disabilities). My mom was a tough advocate for my disability; she knew what I was capable of, that I knew my colors, and believed in my potential. At the meeting, my teacher spoke up to let the team know that I was a little behind schedule when I first started, but I made significant progress and ensured I knew my colors over time. The case was won, and I was able to attend a mainstream school with students with and without disabilities. I was placed in a self-contained and integrated classroom setting for most of my public school journey.

From that moment, I continued to break away from the low expectations and being defined through the labels. So many of these journeys made me question my path and my worth until this day; I felt like my dreams were shattered. However, instead of focusing on my abilities and what I could do, many people focused on my disability and how it limited me. Despite what many say is impossible due to my disability, I continued to dream big. Was not I supposed to keep dreaming big because I "dream big?"

As I entered middle school, I was transitioning again- not only to a new school and building but to a new classroom setting. I would be in a general education setting with only one teacher and over twenty-five students. It was a higher level of learning. Students with disabilities like myself also went to the resource room as a support service.

What is a Resource Room?

❋ ❋ ❋

A resource room is a service where students in general education settings with IEPs can still receive additional support. People with various disabilities can seek assistance from the resource room teacher if they have difficulty understanding assignments given in the classroom or for homework.

I felt like I was in college when I was in sixth grade. Every day, each class went beyond what my brain could process in a day, and when I got home from school, the work did not end there; it continued. Each day, once I was settled in, it was like a second school day, with homework in each subject and classroom assignments that I did not have time to complete during the school day. I thought I was going crazy because I always wanted to finish my work even if I was physically exhausted, especially when I had to do much handwriting. Though I was frustrated with everything going on academically, I pushed through.

My mother tried to reassure me that everything was fine. On the days I could not complete my assignments, she would write a letter to my teacher to understand why I could not complete the homework assignments. It was overwhelming at times, but my teacher would understand why. I never wanted my mother to write those letters because I believed it would be viewed as an excuse. I never wanted my disability to be considered to be an excuse. When my mom noticed my daily frustration and that I was barely making it past sixty-five in grade average, she asked the teacher whether she felt the class was moving too fast for me. The teacher agreed. The next conversation began with the IEP team, where everyone agreed that I should be placed in a self-contained special education class. This did not mean that I was not smart or incapable of learning.

On the contrary, being in a self-contained special education class allowed me to thrive; I would get individualized attention from the teachers and do well. In eighth grade, I thought I could not attend high school, so I planned to go to trade school. However, my teacher saw my potential and encouraged me to go to high school.

It was tricky when I got to high school because when the school bus arrived to pick me up for my first day of high school, the driver informed my mother that the school was not wheelchair-accessible. This was the first time we learned that not all schools are wheelchair-accessible. It was a whole new chapter of my life. Around the same time, doctors told my parents and me that I needed to have major spine surgery to correct my scoliosis as I had a 90-degree curve, a new diagnosis added to the list besides cerebral palsy. After my surgery, I was scared to move my upper body even though doctors said I was fully recovered. After I graduated, my high school expectations were to be placed in a day program for adults with disabilities so I could focus on my physical and occupational therapy goals, but that is not all I could do with my life. There was more to my life than my disability. I wanted to get a job or go to college. The school's support team never thought college was possible until I graduated from high school and went to college despite my disability while still receiving physical and occupational therapy services. Here I am, still breaking barriers.

How Did I Navigate Adulthood as a person with a disability?

✳ ✳ ✳

Adulthood is difficult for anyone, let alone those with disabilities. I turned 18 years old in high school halfway through my senior year.

What did this imply for me? At 18, I struggled to be outspoken when I felt I needed to be heard. I was just trying to find my way through life; I was so overwhelmed with emotions that it got the best of me. I reacted to things that I felt were wrong, and I wanted it my way. It is not that it was either my way or the highway, as my parents would describe my attitude when I spoke my mind, but it was to say I have a voice too, and I have feelings and dreams that no one will take away from me. I graduated high school and saw a whole new world ahead of me. I took a deep breath because I felt so free to explore life beyond the walls I had known for four years. My only free time was on the weekends when I attended programs, groups, and events.

Adulthood, for me, was another chapter I can describe as a blank chapter. There were few opportunities for an inclusive social life that included a diverse group of people. Turning 18 was a starting point to what was to be in adulthood, yet turning 21 just made everything official about adulthood.

I am still learning in my adulthood that I have not hit all the phases of adulthood yet, but I can still educate others on how far I have come. As an adult with a disability, I notice that some people do not take the time to have conversations with me about life beyond how a disability impacts me. However, I know that the same can be said and noticed by other people with disabilities.

I am here to say that people with disabilities are human and desire the same life as people without disabilities. Everyone needs guidance in life, no matter what.

What was "Turning 18" Like for me until Now?

I always wanted my independence, although I know I will always need support. However, I never wanted my disability to be an excuse for why I could not venture out.

Socially, I stayed in my shell. I did not have a social life because I did not have many friends. Note: If this is you, you are not alone. I attended medical appointments alone.

Growing up in a mainstream environment, especially in school, had a lot to do with my development and showed true inclusion, which meant that I had never seen many people like me growing up.

Growing up, I was never eligible for certain services because of my father's "income." So, along the way, I had to advocate with the systems to receive services and benefits such as food stamps and Social Security.

How did I Access my Capabilities?

Kids with disabilities growing up strive to become independent in their way. I get it; this is me. Growing into these phases, experiences, and chapters is much more than I expected. I am someone that's always making progress.

I feel for those whose disabilities limit them; others need to see their abilities as limitless. For example, those who go to appointments with the home attendants who would not support them or even be their voice, sit with us, embrace us, comfort us, and assure us what the reality is plus what real adult life would be.

I have overcome some issues but still struggle with the most, especially at medical appointments, case managers meetings, etc.

Since I turned 18, I have learned to go to my medical appointments, be out in the community and help me through my college days physically with my home attendant or my Direct Support Professional (DSP). Life was all on me. It was difficult to face fears alone without my supporters or my parents, especially when hearing doctors speak and share reports that are sometimes reality but are too much for me to process. Hearing doctors' words let me know what I do not need when trying to explain my wants and needs when I already know what will benefit my life.

A few years ago, I remembered asking one of my doctors for a prescription for physical therapy. The doctor asks,

"Did you fall recently?"

I replied, "No"

She replied, —You do not need a prescription for physical therapy if you were not recently injured.

As a kid, I heard doctors speak strongly about getting physical therapy and moving my body to keep myself in shape.

This doctor was trying to tell me my disability was stable and not going to get better or worse, so I did not need physical therapy; the perception I got was that there was no hope that I could make progress with my abilities.

I recently called the Social Security Administration to ask about letters I received about changes made to my benefits. As soon as I gave the agent my information, she asked me if I had a representative payee. I said, "Yes, my mom is my representative payee". She asked for her name. I gave it to her, and once she processed all of that information, she refused to let me continue to speak because my mom is my representative payee; she can only speak to my mom.

I was speechless. Although my mom is my representative payee, I can still speak for myself. This was just a reminder that I have to continue advocating for so many things, including myself and those who need assistance. Take control of your life and continue to control your voice whenever possible because you never know when it will prevent you from advocating for things in your life.

Take control of your voice even if you do not have confidence in YOUR voice. It is your life that you carry with you each day. These things shaped me into who I am today and made me an advocate for change.

Disability and Adulthood

Everyone experiences transition in many phases of their life, and transition looks different for everyone. When I speak about my high school experiences, I get stuck in a frame that I cannot seem to get out of because I was so "isolated" from the other students, who did not get to know me because those in special education classes were held in a separate section of the school. I had to stay in one school area all day on the first floor. More than half of the day was spent in a box-sized classroom with no vents or windows.

I sometimes wished I could have escaped from the space and become more integrated with my peers and school groups. I received my related services such as occupational therapy (OT) and physical therapy (PT) in the bathroom used for students like me who had different needs to be met throughout the school day because the school did not have a designated room with an open space that would allow moments and therapeutic equipment for those who needed the services. Every day during my four years in high school was so repetitive that I got comfortable. I thought that is what the real world would be like. These days, I see nothing but school, home, and my world filled with challenges. These educational and life assessments never included my dreams, goals, talents, gifts, and plans for the future. So they never really saw that side of me because they never took the time to get to know me. They had a societal definition of people/students with disabilities. The lack of expectations affects me as a student with a disability and my peers without disabilities, who are considered to be from an underserved community; we are not going to make it very far.

In this path of transition, I questioned my worth so much. When you graduate high school, you most likely have an idea of your future. However, I felt hopeless with all my diagnoses and "labels," especially being seen as "limited" due to my physical disability. In June 2013, I began to exceed expectations. I graduated in the top ten of my high school graduating class but was left hopeless about my future because I was left without a plan to either go to college or have a career, while my other peers had plans for after high school. I wondered what was in store for me. I was left to figure it out on my own. The supportive team at my high school had planned on keeping me stuck in my frames or society's frames of a future of a person with a disability. The transition plan process in schools that includes planning my future was supposed to begin earlier in my life, but that was not my situation. The discussion started in my senior year. I feared I would be sitting at home with nothing to do. Transition planning in schools is supposed to begin with working with students starting to plan by the age of 12, then by the ages of 14 to 21 for students with disabilities. When I was transitioning to high school, my eighth-grade teacher told my mom to ensure that she met with the IEP team to ensure that I got a local diploma. At the time, I wondered why that opinion was so important. Unfortunately, this is not always the case for students with disabilities who at the time earned an IEP diploma which provides them a limited opportunity in terms of higher education or career. I was one of those who had to deal with a lack of transition planning, but it earned a local diploma that granted me many pathways to college. When asked about my future planning in my senior year, I did not have much to say, not because I was not interested; I had no idea what opportunities were ahead of me.

It was never a conversation of importance, but I was very aware of the expectations of my related services from a very young age, like physical and occupational therapy, so whenever I did not see the expectations at each session, I would tell my mom. For three and a half years, I had an occupational therapist that I did not like to see each session in high school. I did not approve of the quality of the service. My goals in therapy were always to increase my strength and ability. However, according to the Department of Education and my therapist at that time, that goes for a therapist like occupational, physical, and speech services. The goals transition to "life skills." I felt like I was not reaching my goals of doing hand exercises and was given basic goals like computer skills, something I already knew. Advancing my abilities would allow me to function in society. That is something that will never change about my life.

As a result of my focus and wanting to have the benefits of my services, my school's team of teachers, service providers, and my case manager determined that a day program was the best fit due to my many physical limitations and support needs. That was the only recommendation from my case manager and school IEP team on how they felt it could benefit my life. Conversing with students allows students to feel comfortable having a say or just speaking up about their own lives and plans for their future goes a long way about life goals, dreams, skills assessment, interests, passions, and opportunities.

I feared for weeks that I would be sitting home on the computer and not be as productive with my days by searching the web and being on social media. Transition in my vision should include a transition coordinator and members who have a passion for making a difference in someone's future.

Here is how to develop a successful transition plan

- Do weekly or monthly check-ins with students in transition and schedule meetings about the individual student transition process and plan. Transition is about the individual making it customizable to the student. Transition is not just about placement and what I call a one-size-fits-all approach to "disability."

- Bring the student to the table.

- Students with disabilities deserve opportunities and not just one given path and a system of support within the transition team.

Let us go beyond the basic IEP transition meeting to discover more!

At the end of this process, I never pushed myself to excel in my academics because I earned enough to graduate with a diploma.

To students, your transition plan is about you. The future you are being built. Remember, "there is nothing about you without you."

Transition is a discovery chapter, just like learning. Transition becomes a challenge, especially when age becomes a barrier. Unfortunately, many organizations that support people with disabilities have an age limit requirement, and we no longer have access to those organizations.

We need support and fun for the rest of our life. For people with disabilities, why should age be a barrier to accessing programs such as camps and social and emotional support events that give many people with disabilities and their families a break from their day-to-day life? People with disabilities began to wonder what you or your young adult child would do next.

There is much fear of the unknown in the transition process, especially stepping out into a world or community unprepared to embrace individuals with disabilities.

Transition tip 1

Guidance counsellors should be more involved in the transition process.

Transition tip 2

Start building a network, a community, and a support system that will work you through life on good and bad days.

Transition tip 3

Follow your dreams and goals.

Transition tip 4

Create your path if needed.

Transition tip 5

Do not let societal expectations force you into limiting how far you can go.

Questions about the transition from school

Was there anxiety when you were transitioning from school?

How did the school handle the transition process? Was it easy on your parents?

Was the transition process equal?

How did your parents feel about the transition?

My Path to College

I n college, I felt accepted and welcomed by my peers and educators, Although I was unsure how successful I would be in college.

The financial process, including financial aid and other academic scholarship from state agencies like Adult Career and Continuing Education Services (Access VR) for college, was never confirmed from the start of the college process. I knew I could not afford college from the start, with my dad being the only provider and me not having a job. I always had a goal to do things for myself as much as possible and make mom and dad happy.

Growing up very young, I talked with my parents about becoming a lawyer, but I always hesitated because it required eight years of college or more. However, education has its cost and benefits. I did not want to be on this college path forever. Although I worked hard despite the reality of limitations, I did my best academically. I was never assured of the bright future I could have when I graduated high school.

Students are required to take a second language in high school, but those with IEPs were not required to take it. Why? I have no idea why things are set up that way. So many times, I wondered, *why push to the top? What will I do with my high school diploma when I graduate?*

I wondered if people like me with mobility and physical needs went to college. I require adaptive equipment for my home attendants to provide me with personal care. The summer before college started in the fall of 2013; it was night and days of phone calls and emails to the college, Access- VR, and the home care agency. Nothing or no one was giving me confident answers. Nevertheless, I was taking steps to start. I accepted my seat at CUNY Kingsborough Community College.

My dad accompanied me to take my placement exams on campus. I had no idea what the expectations were for this exam to be prepared and aim to excel at it. I told myself I would do my best and thrive in college. I attended orientation with my mom, and we met with the Director of Disability Services at Kingsborough Community College. She greeted mom and me and recognized I was the student calling every day to ask questions and make sure they were aware of me to attend classes on campus with my unique needs. She took us into a room and sat down with me and my mom and said to me, "tell me what I need to do to accommodate you? I showed the director of Accessibility services the adjustable table that I would need so that My aides could support me with my personal needs. She did not hesitate to take action; she confirmed the funding and placed the order, no questions asked, and told me it would be placed in the nurse's office to go there each time I needed to use the bathroom. I knew then that college was the place for me.

By the fall of 2013, I was ready to enroll in college; whether or not I had my home care attendants to support me days before the first day of class, things were still unsure about getting the okay for extended home care hours. I had already registered for classes and was scheduled to begin them on the first day of the semester. So, I came up with Plan B; like in every situation, a Plan B should be created. I connected with two of my friends who worked with me at a summer day camp formally known as United Cerebral Palsy of New York City (Now it is called Adapt Community Network in Brooklyn) who worked in the field as Direct Support Professionals. So, when I reached out to them to see if they could accompany me to college and support me on campus, they were ready to do it. At that time, I did not have the flexibility to hire my aides. They took me for my first week of classes until my extended home care hours were approved. They kept me encouraged and reminded me never to give up. I thought I would hire them, but to be a self-hire worker, you need to have a strong workers' system to be independent and have reliable workers because what will I do if my aide calls out sick? I cannot depend on my mom and my dad. The college journey was where I put some of my fears aside, as I never wanted to make my situations/obstacles get in my way of achieving all that I am capable of.

Each semester was a story of its own. Each semester involved dealing with self-doubt, questioning if I could do this and get it done. I spent over six years in college.

Outline of Each Year

In the fall of 2013 began my first semester of college at Kingsborough Community College. It was an eye-opening experience for me. First, all of my requested disability accommodations were received. Then, I arrived at each of my classes and saw an accessible student classroom desk that my wheelchair could go under. I have never seen an accessible classroom desk throughout my years in public school.

Nothing was a fight or anything to stress about like it was in my public school. My motto was, "No matter what, I am doing the work and getting it done." Each semester I balanced my classes between the easy and heavy loads. I never took any more than two or three classes a semester. It also depended on the times the classes were offered. My classes had to be scheduled between 10:20a.m and 2:50 pm; so that my aides could leave at 4:30 pm or 5:30 pm. I truly felt confined to a life beyond my control. At my time, I had the support of my aide between 8: 30a.m and 4: 30p.m Monday to Thursday, and one day of the week was until 5:30 pm, and Friday was 10 am to 4 pm. Friday was set for mostly my physical therapy appointments or medical appointments. In my first semester of college, I realized real-life struggles as a young adult with a disability and college student. The main struggle of college was dealing with the Access A Ride issue that truly was never seen much because before, I only used the service for medical appointments. Access A Ride is a paratransit system used to get elderly and People with disabilities around New York City. From the very beginning, they showed they were unreliable, picking me up late, getting me to class late, and often just in time for me to go to my next class. If I had only one class, it would be just 10 minutes before class would end.

My college advisor helped me enroll in my classes each semester and decide what would work best. So, at the very beginning of my college journey, I majored in computer science.

I took remedial English and a college-accredited course at the beginning of my college journey. In the fall of 2013, I started by taking remedial English and Women in American History. I got an A in English and a B in Women in American History. My GPA was a 3.0.

I began to get involved on my college campus from the second semester onward. I was asked to speak on a panel on disability and bullying for a disability-awareness month on campus in April 2014.

This semester, I was accepted to be a part of the National

Honor Society. I had no idea what to do with the invitation. My mom was the one to receive and see the letter. When I saw it, I was surprised.

In the first 2014 spring term, I took another remedial English reading and writing course and History of Phi modern. In English reading/writing, I got an A–. In the History of phi modern, I got a C+. In my second session, I took a speech class in speaking and listening. I do not believe it focused a lot on public speaking, but I got a B.

This was the semester I also finally passed my college reading exam above the grade level. My IEP stated I was on a fifth of sixth-grade level in math or reading.

Spring term 2014 GPA 2.65.

In the fall of 2014, I took CUNY developmental writing and general psychology.

Here is what my grades were:

CUNY developmental writing: B

General psychology: C–

Fall semester GPA: 1.7

At Kingsborough Community College, I was still considered a good academic record, but this could differ from the state agency that funded my college education. I must maintain a GPA of 2.0 or higher. I was still considered in the fifth or sixth level in math or English/reading in high school, so how did I pass my CUNY reading with a few points higher than expected standards?

Here are the courses I took with my grades in the spring 2015 regular session:

Comparative government – A

Intro to sociology – A

The second term session was another history course focusing on Europe napoleon

Europe napoleon – A

Term GPA 4.0. All hard work and determination.

In 2016, I changed my major to liberal arts with a minor in English after realizing computer science requires a lot of math courses—a subject that was never easy for me to process. I could learn, but I got through with the basics. I never wanted to be stuck in the process of learning. I always had that determination to keep on going no matter what.

I was finally able to enroll in college-level English; after passing my CUNY writing exam, I got a B + in English. After not cutting a few times, I decided to try a different technique like hand-writing it without using the computer and passed it.

How did I discover a lot about how I learn and how my brain processes things?

✳ ✳ ✳

Although I switched my major from computer science to liberal arts, I could balance out the courses by taking courses of my interest. I took a computer course that focused on digital photo illustrations, where I learned about Photoshop and editing photos. There, I realized my love for capturing photos and how powerful photos can be with the message that they carry. It was a challenge since I had to use multiple keys on the keyboard to make changes. My professor made things very adaptive for me. He showed me a way to use my other hand to access the other key functions and get my assignments done. As a result, I got an A+ in the course. This is proof that I never let my limitations limit me. In the second semester, I took a Survey of Art History course.

That semester, despite having to leave my art class early to catch a ride on time so my home care worker could end her shift on time, I wondered if I was capturing any knowledge. So I took pictures of the notes on the board provided by the professor using my phone to ensure that I kept up and captured the needed information for that class. I had projects where I had to visit different art museums in NYC, and thankfully, with the support of my community habilitation staff at that time, I was able to make this possible.

My term GPA = 3.33.

I often do not know how I made it happen, but I did. I kept on going no matter what. In the fall of 2016, I enrolled in my second college English course and a basic desktop in publishing, where I learned many skills. I created flyers, menus, business cards, and newsletters and do so even today. I have a passion for using my skills to develop them into my own business one day. This is what I wanted to experience in college; l wanted to learn things and put them to use.

Grades for fall 2016

English course 200 – B+

Basic desktop in publishing – A+

2016 fall term GPA – 3.65

I began to face my struggles and discouragement in silence in the 2017 spring semester as my goal was to thrive no matter the obstacles and demands of my coursework or life that came my way. When I switched my major to liberal arts, I also had a minor concentration in English as I began to discover my passion for working with kids and becoming an educator.

I took three courses that included an introduction to literature, American government, and politics. As an elective, I took career counseling and explored my interest in becoming a teacher's assistant. I told myself I was good enough. In my introduction to literature course, my professor must have noticed me falling behind or feeling discouraged based on my grades and submitting assignments, and he looked at me and said, "You have come so far to give up now; stay focused." That meant everything to me when I needed such encouragement the most. He even scheduled office hours to support me and ensure I completed my assignments and got through the course.

> Intro to Literature – B+
>
> American Government and Politics – A
>
> Career Counseling – A
>
> Term GPA – 3.70

Moreover, when I completed the courses, it felt like a weight was lifted from me. It is amazing how people, especially this professor, noticed I had a lot going on, yet I have potential and determination. No matter how many times I had to correct things to reach the professor's expectations, I knew it would take a long time, and the results have proven it.

When I arrived in the fall 2017 semester, I started breaking down after a few weeks. I truly began to feel drained physically and mentally. I enrolled in three courses that semester: English in Literature, Introduction to Literature Short Fiction, and Strait Gate College Success.

I am self-driven when I see no reason I cannot achieve anything or get things done because of my disability. I enrolled in two English classes, one of which was writing intensive. Each semester, I completed my deadlines and laid out my expectations, allowing me always to make the impossible "possible." While in college, I needed to meet my disability needs, and the opportunities I was given to make a difference motivated me. Mom always told people, "I do not know how Ketrina does it, but she is always ready to make things happen."

Days or weeks into the semester, I rolled into my World Literature class, sitting at my desk, and I just wanted to roll out of the classroom and cry and give up because I was overwhelmed, but I did not. I held it together and started to think of a master plan. How will I get through this semester?

It was all about decisions. Why is it so hard for me to decide on things?

To balance things out:

1. I reached out for support.

2. I talked with the professor and asked her if I could do the work from home and bring it to her; she told me she would ask the department if it was possible.

3. When the professor informed me that it could not be possible, I withdrew from the class. When many asked about the class, the best thing I said was that I did not need that class anymore. I took college work to maintain my GPA.

Here are my grades:

World Literature, Introduction to Literature Short Fiction and Straitgate College Success– B

Introduction to Literature Short Fiction – A

World Literature – W

Term GPA – 3.75

Things just became overwhelming, maintaining life as a young person. Then, in 2016, I got the opportunity to be a volunteer intern through reading partners to tutor kids in reading at NYC public schools. This opportunity centered around my passion for teaching kids, and I received an award from Kingsborough for community service.

During that very semester, I worked with an organization called INCLUDEnyc in a project possibility program that helps young people plan for the future. I was in the process of transferring to a four-year college after talking with an INCLUDEnyc educator about my true passion for being an educator. She told me I could become a special education teacher because I had a very supportive team and a good view of what I will do as an educator. I believe I can do anything. When we reached out to my Access VR counselor to inform her of my plan, I was told that if I transferred to a four-year college, they would be able to continue to fund my college tuition. I went through applying to a four-year college, and in the process, I wanted to give up because the process seemed impossible. However, I kept pushing after a phone call of encouragement from my INCLUDEnyc educator. This girl who never expected to make it this far got accepted to LIU Brooklyn with a merit honor scholarship, but even with the scholarship, it did not cover the full needs of my tuition. Then I got accepted to the CUNY School of Professional Studies Disability Studies Program, which was my dream come true. I was delighted to be in a learning environment surrounded by more than just a next-level education. My interest and passion still surround me, and accessible learning remains because the disability studies program is entirely online.

In January of 2018, I started my Spring 2018 term at CUNY SPS. I enrolled in Biology 200 with a lab and another course in disability and society. I was empowered by the flexibility I had been given to thrive. I started the biology course and had a disability in social class.

Although I was falling behind, I caught up with my biology course and finished my science labs. I eventually got a C in biology.

As a result of an overload in work, I asked my disability and society professor if I could get a grade extension. However, my professor informed me that it was not possible since I needed to complete more than one assignment for the course. In addition, college takes much time, energy, and sleepless nights to push forward.

I accepted a failing grade for the course, and my GPA dropped to its lowest, a 1.0. I was lost, wondering if I would be given a second chance. Access VR already told me that I only had one semester to complete my bachelor's degree since I used up all my allowed semesters toward completing my associate's degree. Does that mean I am not smart enough or capable enough for college? I had to question my intelligence; as a result, how does a program supporting people with disabilities define how long we are expected to take to complete our higher education?

As a result of my GPA dropping to 1.0, I was placed on academic probation. I appealed against it by writing a letter explaining my situation. A few weeks later, I got an email saying my appeal letter was approved. I was thankful to say this journey was meant to be because if the school did not approve the appeal, I would not be able to go back to school. I met with my advisor and enrolled for my bachelor's degree in my second semester. I enrolled in a math course and mental health course. Access VR had already told me that due to my GPA dropping to 1.0, they could not pay for the semester, so I relied on financial aid from the school and the balance. I would have no choice but to use my monthly Social Security income. Days and weeks into the semester, I realized that every time I opened up my computer to work, I would become overwhelmed with emotions and just close the computer or switch the page just to do something different.

Then one day, I completely crashed into emotions and said *I could not do this anymore; today was the day I withdrew from my classes before it was too late.* I think that breakdown happened the day before the deadline to withdraw from classes without having to pay a percentage of the tuition.

Weeks and months into that semester, I went back into my CUNYFirst account and realized my withdrawal from the classes was never processed. That meant I was responsible for the tuition for classes I never completed.

Furthermore, nothing in the system showed I attempted to process the withdrawal at that date and time. I also appealed it with another letter explaining what I was going through and needed to withdraw and take a break from school/classes. That appeal was denied. I submitted proof of my disability. I truly did not know what to do. I felt colleges are not seeing how college can impact a person's physical and mental health, especially young people trying to maintain life, education, medical needs, and beyond. I never imagined going to physical therapy and college simultaneously being so overwhelmed, especially when scheduling my times around my aide's schedule.

When I told my doctors I was going to college in 2013, they reminded me to do what was best for me. However, some of my doctors were proud of me for standing up for myself in this situation, especially since I could not balance out physical therapy and college. I took a year off from college to take care of myself mentally and physically and thrive in opportunities with my continuing reign as Ms. Wheelchair NYS 2018. Ms. Wheelchair New York is a pageant competition that promotes disability awareness, education, and advocacy and celebrates the accomplishments of women who use wheelchairs. In the fall of 2019, I was ready to enroll back in college, and my motto became, "No matter what, I am in it to win." I started this college journey from the beginning. I was ready to prove my intelligence again. I enrolled at Touro College in my area, just a bus ride away. Ready to turn a new page. I enrolled as a full-time student to get financial aid. Although my tuition still cost a lot, I had to make things happen.

Before realizing the missing gaps in special education and general education systems, I got to college. I took the college math placement assessment at Touro College, but I did not pass. This was when I realized I was never taught a wide range of different kinds of math concepts. No matter how many times I looked at this placement exam, trying to figure out the work and do my best, it looked like a foreign language. I started to think I had a math learning disability, not to put another label on myself, but this was a subject I had struggled with since I was in middle and high school. I was taught the basics, as those in special education are taught at a lower level than those in general education in special education self-contained classes. I realized the work was modified, but our teachers taught us less of the topics to make it easier to understand, but at the same time, we were short-changed on what we needed to know.

Then, while at Touro College, it appeared that it would take me a little longer to get my associate's degree because I needed to take a certain number of Touro college credits to earn my associate's degree. It is surreal that I was already so close to finishing my degree and had been through so much that I just wanted to keep that sense of hope alive. I promised to take away, no matter the barriers that come my way. *I am getting this degree.*

Here are my grades from the semester at Touro College

History: A–

Human service: A

Speech and Communication: A

Survey of Mental Health and Disability: F

Term GPA: 2.78

So, does a failing grade make you or me a failure or incapable of succeeding?

I always talk about creating a path to doing things that work best for me to achieve my goal and maintain my interest.

After reaching out to Kingsborough Community College, they shared my possibilities for getting my associate's degree. I learned that the college had a reverse transfer program that allowed me to earn my associate's using two of my credits from my time at Kingsborough Community College and other universities/colleges I attended. I became transparent about my struggles to pass the remedial math assessment. They informed me that if I took an equivalent college math course as a non-degree student and got a C or better, I would be eligible for my associate's degree.

What is Reverse Transfer?

A student who has transferred to a baccalaureate institution from a community college without first earning an Associate's degree might still be able to earn that associate's degree. With a reverse transfer, credits earned at the baccalaureate institution that meet and complete the academic credentials of the associate's degree are "transferred back" from the four-year institution to the two-year institution.

In college, I understood my learning style with what worked and did not achieve and progress in my courses. I learned from the start of college that I do things differently and learn differently. I did many things to help keep me focused.

For example, my folders and notebooks were brightly colored. I frequently copy pages from my textbooks/reading books to highlight and take notes on paper. I felt more connected to the paper. The first time I took the CUNY Reading

Assessment was at the start of my college journey.

The accommodation I had was a reader who gave me a videocassette and headphones to listen to the readings, although I can read and hear things aloud. However, my attention was still all over the place with the cassette because I could not concentrate using recorded audio. So the next time I took it, I told the workers at the Accessibility Department that these headphones did not work for me. I need someone to sit by me and read the texts and passages.

Guess what? As a result of recognizing what works for me, I passed my CUNY Reading Assessment. Just like that, I did it. I recognized how I learned and considered myself a problem solver because I find a way to make it happen no matter what comes my way.

I took my CATW CUNY Writing Test a few times, and once I got an idea of the expectations for this exam, I passed. Each time I typed my essay out on the laptop, I had confidence that I did my best. Nevertheless, I would fail. I continued to question myself. I was doing everything that my professors taught me.

Nevertheless, I was not passing, so I started to think, Is the computer making me *"dumb?"* I thought again; *I would work tirelessly to write my papers by hand and dictate them to my "scribe"* so that my professor could clearly understand the wording. Not because I cannot write neatly, but my words can get too close together, so I like to separate my thoughts.

For the CATW assessment, I wrote it out by hand and then

read it over to my scribe, who wrote it over for me. As I was doing so, I caught my own mistakes and corrected them. I passed the exam with flying colors, exceeding the original grade levels expected.

Then when I got the opportunity to take college math as a non-degree student, I took the course. This was the course I needed to pass to earn my associate's degree. I looked into many different colleges that offered non-degree programs. I enrolled in Penn Foster Math Statistics. A few days into looking through the coursework and textbook, I felt discouraged and said, *I do not know this stuff.* I was so frustrated that I dis-enrolled immediately and started college-level math at SUNY Empire State College. I made my situation known, and my professor encouraged me from the start of the semester. At the beginning of the semester, I struggled again.

I would look at my math workbook each day and close it because I could not seem to process the information independently. The math language seemed far away and had no connection. I felt like I could not learn this. I would break down into tears often. My dad encouraged me each day during the nights and weekends and told me I should not beat myself up for this. He supported me, working through the math problems with me. The intensity of the courses was the first thing I noticed after enrolling in college, so I decided to contact Disability Services and request "accommodations." Accommodations paved the way for me to excel in my courses. The extended time on home assignments and extended tutoring sessions helped me improve academically.

Although in the beginning, I felt like I was falling behind weeks, when my professor noticed my willingness to be productive in the course but was still falling behind, she recommended a tutor who specialized in the math course I was taking. From that moment, things took off for the better every day. For almost two to three hours a day, I would attend live tutoring sessions on Zoom.

The tutoring process was a miracle because I was able to get through the semester, and in this math course, I had three different tutors help me. Then, in the evenings and at night, I used smart thinking 24/7 tutoring services to complete my coursework between 10 am and 11 pm. My caregivers, my parents, were awake during the night. Leaving this in my college life to be confined and go beyond my control. My tutors guided me through my math assignments so that I could understand and process them step by step. This was when I realized that I knew math but had never been able to process it independently as a whole through a big picture.

Once I did things step-by-step, I was able to respond with my answers and share my knowledge of understanding at the moment, whether I remember the process or not. It got me through my assignments, and when I talked through the steps with the tutors, I was proud of myself. Whenever I made errors on assignments, I would always make an effort to correct my mistakes to balance out my grades.

My professor offered to support me, and even after the tutoring sessions with my tutors, my tutor offered to help me.

She would even call me on the weekend to go through my

assignments with me. After excelling at my discussion boards with my classmates and passing my classwork assignments, I saw the light at the end of the tunnel.

After 15 weeks into the semester, I did it. I took my math final and got a 70 of 100 on it. In this whole process, I shocked myself that I had made it this far. The one who struggled with math all her life in school and even in college got an A in college math from SUNY Empire State College. From then, I began transferring my credits back over to Kingsborough Community College to be processed by the Reverse Transfer Program. By May 2020, my associate's degree was awarded through the Reverse Transfer Program.

In June 2020, I graduated with my associate's degree in general liberal arts with honors. I am a true miracle trailblazer because no matter what came my way, I paved the way to achieve my plan to graduate college. I truly discovered that my intelligence in college exceeded so many expectations, especially within the level of education stated on documents such as my IEP. As stated on my IEP, I was on a fifth- or sixth-grade level in math or English. I was always considered grade levels behind due to my lack of academic confidence, which limited me from doing great things. I wish that educators in my school system at the time recognized that. If an educator had recognized that, how much potential would they have noticed instead of imposing so many limitations on me and others with IEPs? I pose a question here: What can you do as educators in the school system to help me overcome my lack of confidence and build me up? There is a School-Based Support Team in schools where teachers provide support by recommending classroom- based interventions for students who are struggling academically and behaviorally. This is a question for you to think about for parents and educators. Do all schools have a strong School-Based Support Team that will allow the students to reach their full potential with support? If not, this is where you can advocate for your child. Only 6% to 7% of students with disabilities graduate from college. Along the line, I began to question why I was in college. I felt like what I was learning was never relevant to my interests. However, in my English classes, I was always able to make an interesting connection by sharing my story and experiences. None of the courses were competent enough to prepare me for the real world. I expected the courses to prepare me with knowledge and skills for my career, but this was not always the case. Despite my other struggles in college, I worked hard. I was inducted into many honor societies and was honored to participate in each induction and celebration. In June 2014, I was inducted into the National Society Leadership and Success. My parents got to attend my induction events and dinners. They were proud of my academic achievements, and they still often speak about these memories, and they were elated that the college saw me as a person beyond my disability. What a difference between the high school, where I was frequently forgotten among my peers, and college, where I heard my name called to receive my award among my peers. I appreciate college for being inclusive and accepting!

In January 2018, I was inducted into the Society for Collegiate Leadership and Achievement.

In February 2018, I accepted to be inducted into another honor society called the "Chi Alpha Epsilon Delta Phi Chapter."

In May 2020, I was inducted to be a member of the honor society organization. Society often defines success as a person with a college degree, a house, and a good job; for me, my motto is: "Success is when you follow what your heart desires." Live up to your vision of the American dream.

I faced so many obstacles in college and still made away. However, I often forgot to pause and celebrate my achievements and how I felt to be included as part of the college community.

What was it like for me to participate in student programs like this on campus?

I applied to be a part of the Kingsborough Community College Student Ambassador Program and got accepted in 2017! As a student ambassador, I got a chance to represent my college by attending events and helping out, even at graduation. As part of the student ambassador training, I got to take part in a student ambassador retreat for a weekend at Great Wolf Lodge. So many thoughts started rolling through my head, like: *will I get the chance to be a part of something like this?* As soon as I agreed to be a part of this, my college's Director and Assistant Director of Student Life jumped on board to get approval from the Director of Accessibility and learn the next steps in terms of paperwork and accommodations that I needed to attend. I needed my parents to attend to support me in my physical needs. The director of

Accessibility and Student life ensured that the college would approve my parents to attend due to liability reasons. The Director of Accessibility was pleased that I was involved in a campus student program that was not limited to students with disabilities. She always encouraged students with disabilities to get involved on campus. I was granted permission to attend the weekend retreat. They ordered an accessible coach bus after learning about the accommodations I needed to attend, especially under the ADA (Americans with Disability Act). When I got to the retreat location, the resort had an accessible bus to take me to and from my suite whenever I needed to go to an area on the resort. I even got to do an activity that was considered a safe space activity at one of the other suites that were not wheelchair accessible. The director of the student ambassador program and my peers ensured that they had a way for me to attend. My dad brought me over to the suite to assist me with transferring, and they had a couch set for me with pillows for me to sit up and feel comfortable sitting near me to make sure I did not fall, and I will be okay. They then came back to my suite, bought pizza, and enjoyed a game night with me. My suite had an accessible ramp for easy access. My suite was on the first floor. Every activity on the retreat was made adapted to my abilities. My peers sat and had conversations with me during mealtime. My peers were also welcoming to my parents and understanding of my situation. What I appreciate the most about this experience because I was treated equally despite my disability.

A World of Doubts

*A*m I doing what makes me happy? Am I taking care of myself? These are things that I should have thought about and advocated for instead of thinking about how others would view me as unsuccessful if I did not complete college. Instead, I stayed in my little world. I felt confined, and college became more of a demand and required all of my focus. I did not have time to hang out with my friends. I could not attend physical therapy because the times available did not fit into my schedule. I had my home attendant's support, and truly my body felt ready to get moving, yet I had to stop going. I was sad not being able to make way for physical therapy, knowing that doctors would prefer me to do physical therapy as it help to keep my muscles moving. I felt as if I had put my life on hold to pursue higher education.

When I received my associate's degree with honors in June 2020, I knew I was in for a whole new chapter once I graduated college, and that is when I felt so free and started living limitlessly. No one can get between me and my dreams, and I promised to enjoy life and do what is best for me.

Tips to College Educators

- College educators should meet students with disabilities where they are and keep them encouraged.

- Create an environment in the classroom.

- Treat students with disabilities the same as peers without disabilities and recognize that not all disabilities are visible, so keep the accommodations in mind.

- Check-in with the students with disabilities and offer office hours to allow you to check in with them or for the student to reach out to you. This would make it easier for students to feel confident in asking for help.

- Alternate learning materials in a way that benefits students while maintaining the exact expectations of those who do not have accommodations.